2nd edition, 2014
Mr. H. Roberts
The Netherlands

Table of Contents

SECTION I

QUICK REFERENCE CHARTS

Chapter 1: Washing your hands

Hygiene is of utmost importance, especially before, during and after applying first aid care. It is important, because you want to minimize cross-contamination. Therefore, keep the following simple steps in mind, to ensure that you wash your hands in the correct manner:

Wet your hands with warm, not hot water

1 Preferably not too hot or too cold.

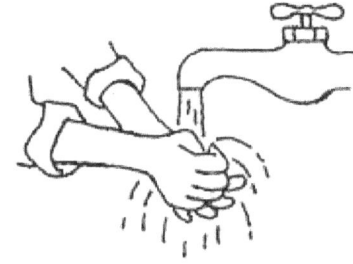

Apply disinfectant soap and scrub hands

2 Rub and scrub your hands extensively for at least 20 seconds. Make sure to cover all parts of your hands and wrists, and pay close attention to fingernails and your rings.

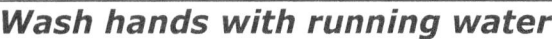

Wash hands with running water

3 Wash your hands with clean, warm water.

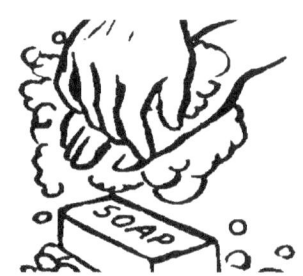

Dry hands preferably with a paper towel

4 Preferably, use a single use, disposable paper towel, and dry thoroughly.

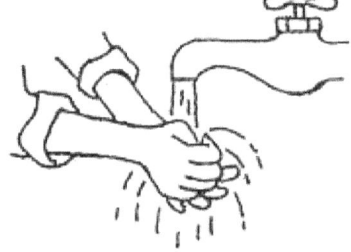

Turn off the water tap with paper towel

5

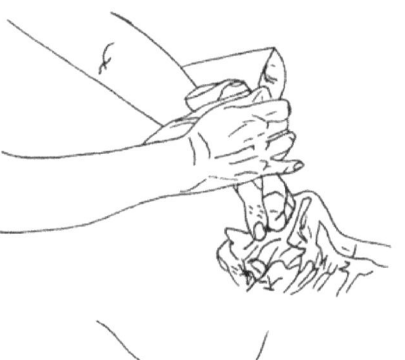

Tips and Tops: Washing your hands

❖ No nailbrush? Scrub jour nails against your palm.

❖ Where possible, use a liquid, disinfectant soap.

❖ When no soap and water is available: use an alcohol based hand sanitizer.

❖ If no paper towel is available, wave and flap your hands in midair until dry.

❖ Preferably, do not use an hot air dryer[1]

Tips and Tops: When to wash your hands?

❖ Before **and** after performing first aid

❖ Immediately after contact with body fluids such as saliva, blood, and others

❖ Before **and** after preparing or handling food

❖ After using the restroom

Notes:

---

[1] Various studies show that a hot air dryer increase the amount of germs in air.

Chapter 2: Checking an injured or ill person

AFTER CHECKING THE SCENE FOR SAFETY, CHECK THE PERSON:

1   *CHECK FOR RESPONSIVENESS*

Tap the shoulder and shout, "Are you OK?"

2   *CALL EMT ...*

If no response, CALL the local emergency number. If an unconscious person is face-down, roll face-up, supporting the head, neck and back in a straight line.

If the person responds, obtain consent and CALL the local emergency number for any life-threatening conditions. CHECK the person from head to toe and ask questions to find out what happened.

3   *OPEN THE AIRWAY*

Tilt head, lift chin.

4   *CHECK FOR BREATHING*

CHECK quickly for breathing for no more than 10 seconds.
■■ Occasional gasps are not breathing.

5   *QUICKLY SCAN FOR SEVERE BLEEDING*

Give CARE based on conditions found.
■IF NO BREATHING—Go to Chapter 4 or 5
(if an AED is immediately available).

■IF BREATHING—Maintain an open airway and monitor for any changes in condition.

Tips and Tops:

- ❖ Use disposable gloves and other personal protective equipment and obtain consent whenever giving care.

- ❖ Write down the local emergency number here….

Notes:

Chapter 3: Choking while Conscious

When food or a foreign object becomes stuck in the throat, it is a scary situation for the person involved, and even potentially life threatening, because it blocks the flow of air. The person will be conscious at first, although not able to speak, breathe, cough or cry. If not acting fast enough, the person will turn unconscious. This chart is based upon the Red Cross "five-and-five" approach. **Note** that treatment for an obese, pregnant or child less than a year is **different!**

Confirm that choking is cause of distress

1 Look for telltale signs such as the person's hands on his neck, bluish lips, or failed attempts to speak.

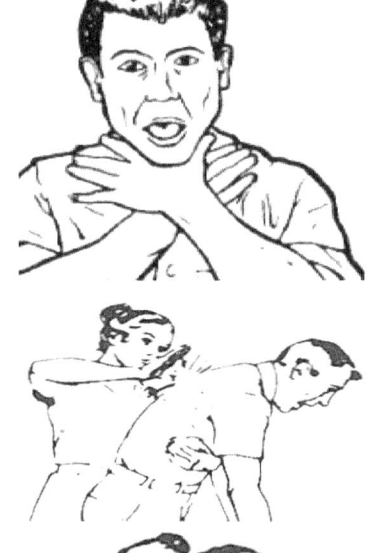

Deliver 5 blows at the back with our palm

2 Strike right between the shoulder blades

Give 5 abdominal thrusts (Heimlich)

3 Stand behind persons and wrap your arms around waste. Make a fist with 1 hand and hold tightly with the other. Lean the victim forward, and give powerful thrusts slightly upwards.

Repeat step 2 and 3

4 Repeat until either the object is forced out or person begins coughing. Stop when person is unconscious.

When person is unconscious

5 Stop directly, carefully lay down the person, and begin to look for the object. Let someone

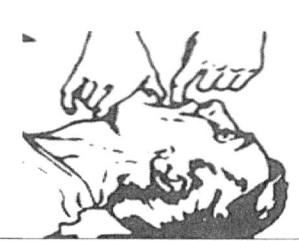

else call the emergency service.

Begin CPR (see next chapter) until paramedics arrive
Tips and Tops: Choking

❖ Ask another person to call the emergency service if possible. Immediate treatment to a conscious choking persons has preference over calling.

❖ If you are physically not able to perform a Heimlich maneuver, please ask someone else to perform.

Tips and Tops: Pregnant & Obese persons

❖ Pregnant and obese persons require a different approach.

❖ You should not aim for the waist during the Heimlich maneuver.

❖ Instead, search the breastbone, and place your hands just below it.

Tips and Tops: Children less than 1 year old

❖ See Chapter 4

Notes:

Chapter 4: CPR – NO BREATHING

AFTER CHECKING THE SCENE AND THE INJURED OR ILL PERSON:

GIVE 30 CHEST COMPRESSIONS

1 Push hard, push fast in the middle of the chest at least 2 inches deep and at least 100 compressions per minute

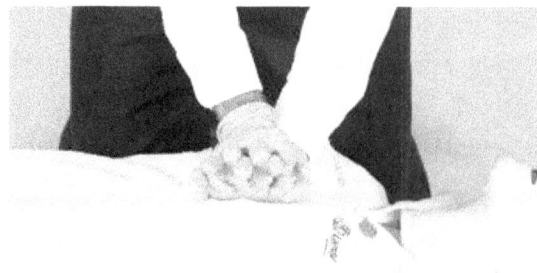

GIVE 2 RESCUE BREATHS

2
■■ Tilt the head back and lift the chin up.
■■ Pinch the nose shut then make a complete
seal over the person's mouth.
■■ Blow in for about 1 second to make the
chest clearly rise.
■■ Give rescue breaths, one after the other.
Note: If chest does not rise with rescue breaths,
retilt the head and give another rescue breath.

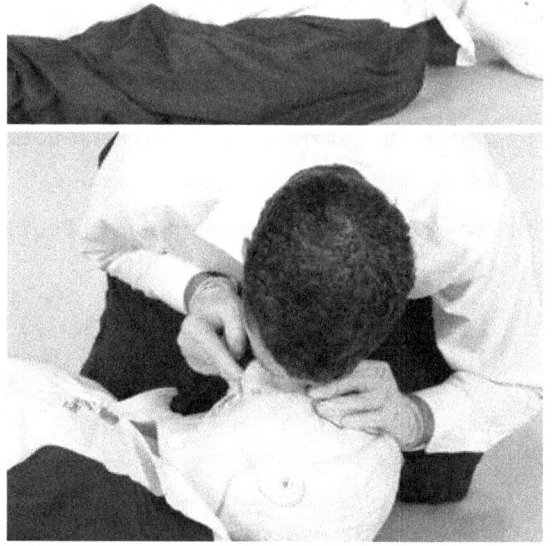

DO NOT STOP

3 Continue cycles of CPR. Do not stop CPR except in one of these situations:
■■ You find an obvious sign of life, such as breathing.
■■ An AED is ready to use.
■■ Another trained responder or EMS personnel take over.

■■ You are too exhausted to continue.

■■ The scene becomes unsafe.

WHAT TO DO NEXT:

IF AN AED BECOMES AVAILABLE—Go to AED, Chapter 5.

IF BREATHS DO NOT MAKE THE CHEST RISE— AFTER RETILTING HEAD—Go to Unconscious choking, Chapter 6.

Tips and Tops:

❖ Person must be on firm, flat surface

❖ If at any time you notice an obvious sign of life, stop CPR and monitor

breathing and for any changes in condition.

Skill Components	Adult	Child	Infant
HAND POSITION	Two hands in center of chest (on lower half of sternum)	Two hands in center of chest (on lower half of sternum)	Two or three fingers in center of chest (on lower half of sternum, just below nipple line)
CHEST COMPRESSIONS RESCUE BREATHS	At least 2 inches Until the chest clearly rises (about 1 second per breath)	About 2 inches Until the chest clearly rises (about 1 second per breath)	About 1½ inches Until the chest clearly rises (about 1 second per breath)
CYCLE	30 chest compressions and 2 rescue breaths	30 chest compressions and 2 rescue breaths	30 chest compressions and 2 rescue breaths
RATE	30 chest compressions in about 18 seconds (at least 100 compressions per minute)	30 chest compressions in about 18 seconds (at least 100 compressions per minute)	30 chest compressions in about 18 seconds (at least 100 compressions per minute)

Notes:

Chapter 5: AED—ADULT OR CHILD

OLDER THAN 8 YEARS OR WEIGHING MORE THAN 55 POUNDS

AFTER CHECKING THE SCENE AND THE INJURED OR ILL PERSON:

1 *TURN ON AED*

Follow the voice and/or visual prompts

2 *WIPE BARE CHEST DRY*

3 *ATTACH PADS*

4 *STAND CLEAR*

Make sure no one, including you, is touching the person.
■■ Say, "EVERYONE, STAND CLEAR."

5 *ANALYZE HEART RHYTHM*

6 *DELIVER SHOCK*

If SHOCK IS ADVISED:
■■ *Make sure no one, including you, is touching the person.*
■■ *Say, "EVERYONE, STAND CLEAR."*
■■ *Push the "shock" button, if necessary.*

7 *PERFORM CPR*

After delivering the shock, or if no shock is advised:
■■ *Perform about 2 minutes (or 5 cycles) of*

CPR.
■■ *Continue to follow the prompts of the AED.*

WHAT TO DO NEXT:

If at any time you notice an obvious sign of life, stop CPR and monitor breathing and for any changes in condition.

Tips and Tops:

- Do not use pediatric AED pads or equipment on an adult or child older than 8 years or weighing more than 55 pounds.
- Remove any medication patches with a gloved hand
- ❖ If two trained responders are present, one should perform CPR while the second responder operates the AED.
- ❖ If at any time you notice an obvious sign of life, stop CPR and monitor breathing and for any changes in condition.

Notes:

Chapter 6: UNCONSCIOUS CHOKING

CHEST DOES NOT RISE WITH RESCUE BREATHS
AFTER CHECKING THE SCENE AND THE INJURED OR ILL PERSON:

GIVE RESCUE BREATHS

1 Retilt the head and give another rescue breath.

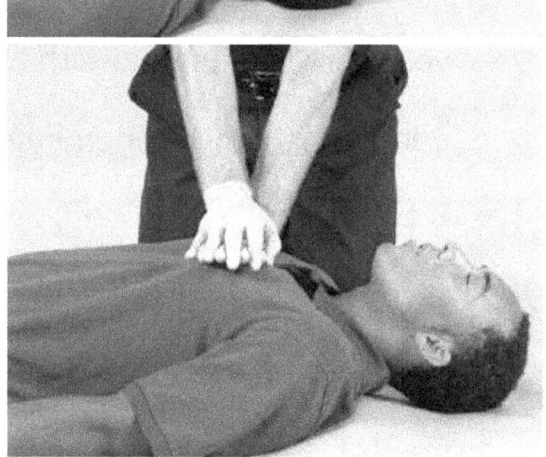

GIVE 30 CHEST COMPRESSIONS

2 If the chest still does not rise, give 30 chest compressions.

LOOK FOR AND REMOVE OBJECT IF SEEN

3

GIVE 2 RESCUE BREATHS

4 Repeat until either the object is forced out or person begins coughing. Stop when person is unconscious.

WHAT TO DO NEXT

5 IF BREATHS DO NOT MAKE THE CHEST RISE—Repeat steps 2 through 4.
IF THE CHEST CLEARLY RISES—CHECK

_____ for breathing. Give CARE.

Tips and Tops:

- ❖ Person must be on firm, flat surface.

- ❖ Remove CPR breathing barrier when giving chest compressions.

Notes:

Chapter 7: CONTROLLING EXTERNAL BLEEDING

AFTER CHECKING THE SCENE AND THE INJURED OR ILL PERSON:

1   *COVER THE WOUND*

Cover the wound with a sterile dressing

---

2   *APPLY DIRECT PRESSURE UNTIL BLEEDING STOPS*

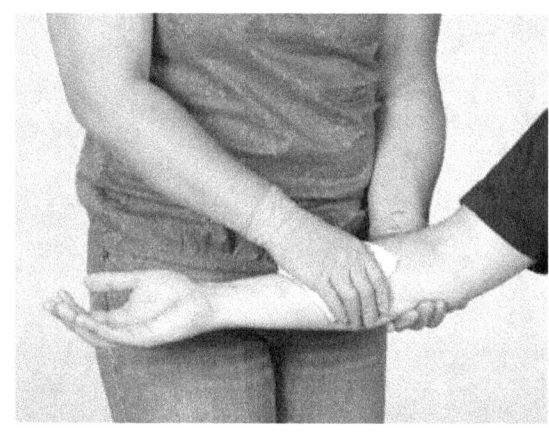

---

3   *COVER THE DRESSING WITH BANDAGE*

Check for circulation beyond the injury (check for feeling, warmth and color).

---

4   *APPLY MORE PRESSURE AND CALL EMT*

If the bleeding does not stop:
- Apply more dressings and bandages.
- Continue to apply additional pressure.
- Take steps to minimize shock.
- CALL EMT or the local emergency number if not already done.

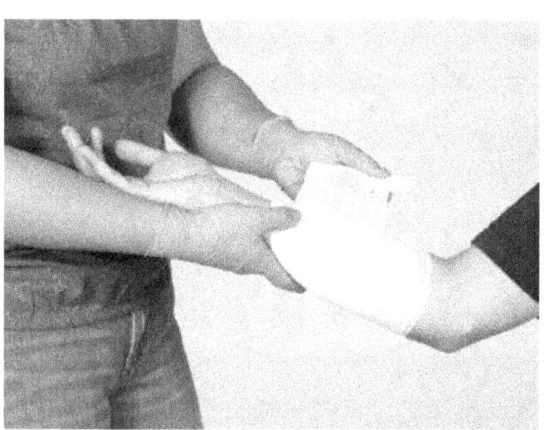

---

5   *WHAT TO DO NEXT*

IF BREATHS DO NOT MAKE THE CHEST RISE—Repeat steps 2 through 4.

IF THE CHEST CLEARLY RISES—CHECK

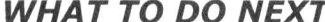

for breathing. Give CARE based on
conditions found.

Tips and Tops:

- Wash hands with soap and water after giving care (See Chapter 1)

Notes:

Chapter 8: BURNS

AFTER CHECKING THE SCENE AND THE INJURED OR ILL PERSON:

1 *REMOVE FROM SOURCE OF BURN*

Cover the wound with a sterile dressing

---

2 *COOL THE BURN*

Cool the burn with cold running water at least
until pain is relieved.

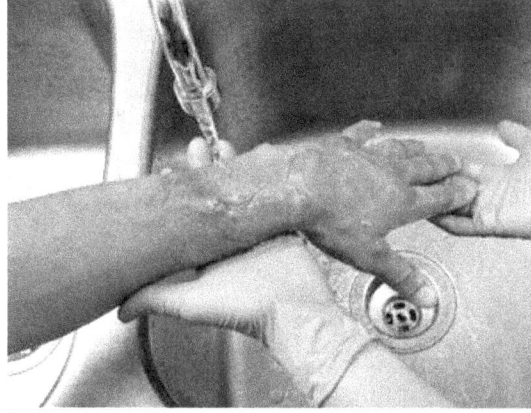

---

3 *COVER LOOSELY WITH STERILE DRESSING*

Check for circulation beyond the injury (check for feeling, warmth and color).

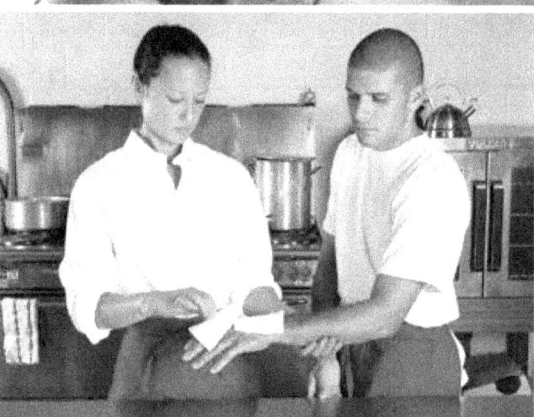

---

4 *CALL EMT*

CALL the local emergency number if the burn is severe or other life-threatening conditions are found.

CARE FOR SHOCK

5

Tips and Tops:

❖ If available, use a burnshield dressing.

Notes:

Chapter 9: POISONING

AFTER CHECKING THE SCENE AND THE INJURED OR ILL PERSON:

CALL EMT OR POISON CONTROL HOTLINE

1 For life-threatening conditions (such as if the person is unconscious or is not breathing, or if a change in the level of consciousness occurs), CALL the local emergency number.
OR
If the person is conscious and alert, CALL the local Poison Control Center hotline and follow the advice given.

PROVIDE CARE

2 Give CARE based on the conditions found

Tips and Tops:

Notes:

Chapter 10: HEAD, NECK OR SPINAL INJURIES

AFTER CHECKING THE SCENE AND THE INJURED OR ILL PERSON:

1 *CALL THE LOCAL EMERGENCY NUMBER*

2 *MINIMIZE MOVEMENT*

Minimize movement of the head, neck and spine.

3 *STABILIZE HEAD*

Manually stabilize the head in the position in which it was found.
■■ Provide support by placing your hands on both sides of the person's head.
■■ If head is sharply turned to one side, DO NOT move it.

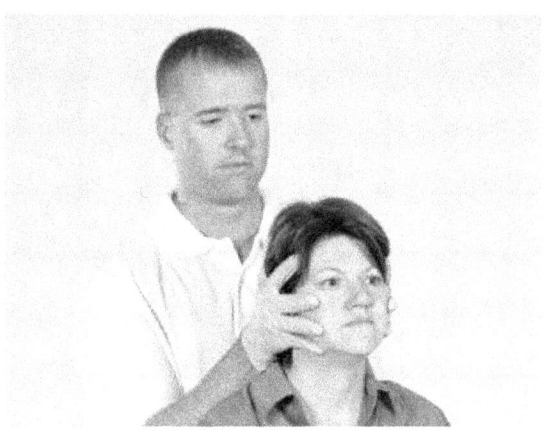

Tips and Tops:

❖ No If available, use a neck collar or spinal board.

Notes:

Chapter 11: STROKE FOR A STROKE, THINK F.A.S.T.

AFTER CHECKING THE SCENE AND THE INJURED OR ILL PERSON:
THINK F.A.S.T.

1

Face— Ask the person to smile. Does one side of face droop?

Arm— Ask the person to raise both arms. Does one arm drift downward?

Speech— Ask the person to repeat a simple sentence (such as, "The sky is blue."). Is the speech slurred? Can the person repeat the sentence correctly?

Time— CALL EMT immediately if you see any signals of a stroke. Try to determine the time when signals first appeared. Note the time of onset of signals and report it to the call taker or EMS personnel when they arrive.

2

PROVIDE CARE

Tips and Tops:

OTHER TELLTALE SIGNS:

- ❖ Sudden numbness or weakness of the face, arm or leg, especially on one side of the body
- ❖ Sudden confusion, trouble speaking or understanding
- ❖ Sudden trouble seeing in one or both eyes
- ❖ Sudden trouble walking, dizziness, loss of balance or coordination
- ❖ Sudden, severe headache with no known cause

Notes:

Chapter 12: REMOVING GLOVES

AFTER GIVING CARE AND MAKING SURE TO NEVER TOUCH THE BARE SKIN
WITH THE OUTSIDE OF EITHER GLOVE:

PINCH GLOVE

Pinch the palm side of one glove
near the wrist.

1

Carefully pull the glove off so that
it is inside out.

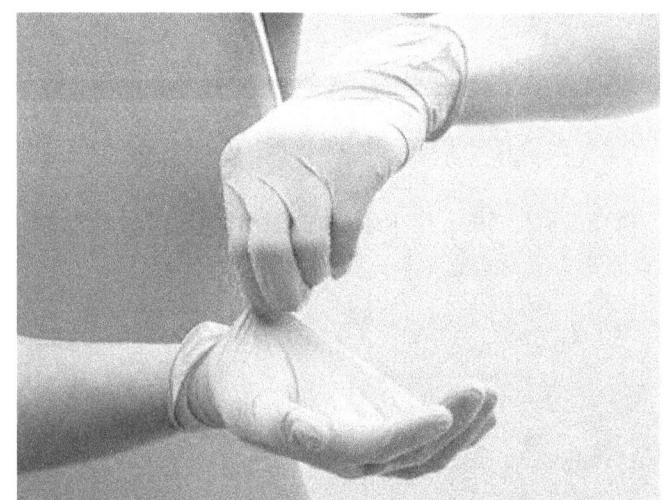

SLIP TWO FINGERS UNDER GLOVE

Hold the glove in the palm of the
remaining gloved hand.

2

Slip two fingers under the glove
at the wrist of the remaining
gloved hand.

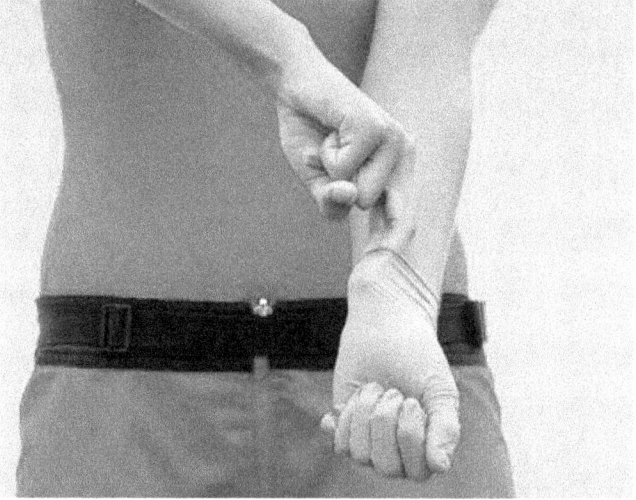

PULL GLOVE OFF

Pull the glove until it comes off,
inside out,
so that the first glove ends up
inside the glove just removed.

3

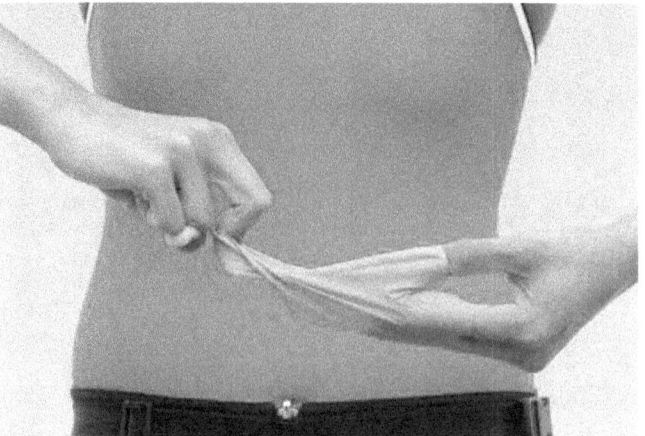

DISPOSE OF GLOVES AND WASH HANDS

After removing the gloves:

4

- Dispose of gloves in the appropriate biohazard container.

- Wash hands thoroughly with soap and warm running water, if available.

- Otherwise, use an alcohol-based hand sanitizer to clean the hands if they are not visibly soiled

Notes:

Chapter 13: USING A MANUFACTURED TOURNIQUET

A Always follow standard precautions and follow manufacturer's instructions when applying a tourniquet. Call the local emergency number.

1 *POSITION THE TOURNIQUET*

Place the tourniquet around the limb, approximately 2 inches (about two finger widths) above the wound but not over a joint.

2 *PULL STRAP THROUGH BUCKLE*

Route the tag end of the strap through the buckle, if necessary.
Pull the strap tightly and secure it in place.

3 *TWIST THE ROD*

Tighten the tourniquet by twisting the rod until the fl ow of bleeding stops and secure the rod in place.
Do not cover the tourniquet with clothing.

4 *RECORD TIME*

Note and record the time that you applied the tourniquet and give this information to EMS personnel

SECTION II

Detailed Information

ASSESSING THE SITUATION

What to Treat First

1. **Don't panic**. You will be able to assess the situation more effectively. Remember, psychological support is also important.

2. **Remember the ABCs of Life Suppor**t:

Airways open – Open and maintain victim's airway.

Breathing restored – If victim is not breathing, begin rescue breathing techniques immediately.

Circulation maintained – If no pulse is present, get assistance from a person certified in cardiopulmonary resuscitation (CPR) techniques.

REMEMBER, to be able to perform CPR effectively, it is essential to be properly trained.

3. **Check for bleeding**. Apply direct pressure and elevate injured limb.

4. **Look for signs of shock and broken bones (fractures)**.

5. **Check for emergency medical identification on the victim**.

6. **Get professional medical help quickly**. Know emergency numbers, such as 0 or 911. Telephone appropriate authorities (rescue squad, ambulance, police, poison control center or fire department) and describe the problem. Be sure to give your name, location and the number of persons involved.

7. **Loosen any clothing** that may restrict victim's breathing or interfere with circulation.

8. Never give an unconscious person anything by mouth.

9. **DO NOT move injured persons** unless situation is life-threatening. Keep victim still, quiet and warm (except heat exhaustion and sunstroke). Victims with broken bones (fractures) should not be moved until a splint has been properly applied.

BURNS & SCALDS

CAUTION

DO NOT clean burns or break blisters. DO NOT remove any clothing that sticks to burn. DO NOT apply grease, ointment or medication to a severe burn. DO NOT use cotton or material with loose fibers to cover burns.

TREATMENT

First degree burns – redness or discoloration of skin surface; mild swelling and pain.
1. Apply cool, wet cloths or immerse in water. DO NOT use ice.
2. Blot gently; apply a dry, sterile pad if necessary.
3. Usually medical treatment is not necessary; however, if severe exist, call for professional medical help. Be alert for signs of shock.

Second degree burns – deep burn with red or mottled appearance; blisters; considerable pain and
swelling; skin surface appears wet. See treatment for first degree burns. If arms and legs are affected,
elevate above heart level. Burns may be deep and potentially serious, requiring medical treatment
depending on extent and location. Be alert for signs of shock and infection.

Third degree burns – deep tissue destruction with a white or charred appearance; no pain. Call for
professional medical help immediately. Be alert for signs of shock.

CUTS & SCRAPES

BEFORE INITIATING ANY FIRST AID TO CONTROL BLEEDING, BE SURE TO WEAR HEALTH CARE GLOVES TO AVOID CONTACT OF THE VICTIM'S BLOOD WITH YOUR SKIN.

1. **CLEAN...** wound and surrounding area gently with mild soap and rinse. Blot dry with sterile pad or clean dressing.
2. **TREAT...** to protect against contamination.
3. **PROTECT...** and cover to absorb fluids and prevent further contamination. (Handle only the edges of sterile pads or dressings.) Secure with first aid tape to help keep out dirt and germs.

SPLINTERS

Slender Pieces of Wood, Bone, Glass or Metal Objects that Lodge In or Under Skin

SYMPTOMS
May Include: Pain, redness, swelling

TREATMENT

1. First wash your hands thoroughly, then gently wash affected area with mild soap and water.
2. Sterilize needle or tweezers by boiling for 10 minutes; wipe with a sterile pad before use.
3. Loosen skin around splinter with needle; use tweezers to remove splinter. If splinter breaks or is
deeply lodged, consult professional medical help.
4. Cover with adhesive bandage or sterile pad, if necessary.

STINGS

CAUTION
In highly sensitive persons, do not wait for symptoms to appear. Get professional medical help immediately. If breathing difficulties occur, start rescue breathing techniques; if pulse is absent, begin CPR.

SIGNS
Signs of allergic reaction may include: Nausea; severe swelling; breathing difficulties; bluish face, lips and fingernails; shock or unconsciousness.

TREATMENT
1. For mild or moderate symptoms, wash with soap and cold water. Remove stinger or venom sac with tweezers or by gently scraping with fingernail (DO NOT squeeze).
2. For multiple stings, soak affected area in cool bath. Add one tablespoon of baking soda per quart of water.

BLEEDING

BEFORE INITIATING ANY FIRST AID TO CONTROL BLEEDING, BE SURE TO WEAR HEALTH CARE GLOVES TO AVOID CONTACT OF THE VICTIM'S BLOOD WITH YOUR SKIN.

TREATMENT
1. **Act quickly**. Have victim lie down. Elevate injured limb higher than heart unless you suspect a broken bone.
2. **Control bleeding by applying direct pressure on the wound** with a sterile pad or clean cloth.
3. **If bleeding is controlled by direct pressure**, bandage firmly to protect wound. Check pulse to be sure bandage is not too tight.
4. **If bleeding is not controlled by use of direct pressure**, apply a tourniquet only as a last resort.
5. Call for professional medical help immediately.

6. **If you are bleeding and have no one to help you**, call for professional medical help.
Lie down, so your body weight applies pressure to the bleeding site.

BREATHING PROBLEMS

ESTABLISH NON-RESPONSIVENESS AND ACTIVATE EMERGENCY MEDICAL SERVICES (EMS) OR CALL FOR HELP.

SYMPTOMS
May include: Shortness of breath, dizziness, chest pain, rapid pulse, bluish-purple skin color, dilated pupils, unconsciousness.

TREATMENT
For victim who has stopped breathing:

1. Lay victim flat on back. Tilt the head back with one hand to open airway, while placing two fingers of the other hand under the chin.
2. Clear airway, using your fingers in a hooked fashion to remove any solid or liquid obstructions.
3. Look, listen, and feel for respiratory movement for 5 seconds. If breathing is absent, pinch victim's nostrils closed, take a deep breath, completely cover victim's mouth, and give two slow, full breaths.
4. Check for carotid pulse in neck and for signs of breathing.
5. If pulse is present:
For adults – continue rescue breathing at a rate of one strong every five seconds. Re-check for pulse and breathing every twelve breaths.
For infants and small children – breathe shallow breaths at a rate of one every three seconds or 20 per minute.
6. If pulse is not present, begin Cardiopulmonary Resuscitation (CPR).
For adults... Exert enough pressure to depress the breastplate 1 1/2 to 2 inches. Continue compressions at a rate of "one and two and..." Every fifteen compressions should be followed with a pause by two rescue breaths.
For children... Use the heel of only one hand to depress the breastplate 1 to 1 1/2 inches. Continue compressions at a rate of 100 per minute "one, two, three..." Every five compressions should be followed without a pause by one rescue breath.
For infants... Use only fingertips. Apply moderate pressure to depress breastplate 1/2 to 3/4 inches. Continue compressions at a rate of at least 100 per minute. Every five compressions (3 seconds) should be followed without a pause by one rescue breath.

BROKEN BONE (FRACTURE)

Break or Crack in a Bone

SYMPTOMS

May include: The victim hearing or feeling the bone break; area tender to touch with pain in one spot;
swelling noted around suspected fracture; limb in an unnatural position; painful movement; abnormal motion; loss of function; grating sensation; discoloration of affected area.

TREATMENT

1. Keep victim warm and still, treat for shock if necessary. **DO NOT move victim until a splint has been applied** unless there is danger of a life-threatening emergency.

2. **If bone is suspected to be broken but does not pierce the skin** (closed fracture), splint the limb before the victim is moved, immobilizing the joint above and below the suspected fracture site.

3. **If broken bone pierces the skin** (open or compound fracture), apply pressure to appropriate pressure point to control bleeding. DO NOT try to straighten limb, return it to a natural position, or replace bone fragments. DO NOT touch or clean the wound. Secure a sterile pad or clean cloth firmly in place over the wound and tie with strong bandages or cloth strips.

4. If victim **must** be moved, apply a splint to prevent further damage. Use anything that will keep the broken bones from moving, including broomsticks, boards or rolled magazines. Pad splints with cotton, clothes or clean cloths tied firmly (but not tightly) in place. If victim complains of numbness, loosen splint.

5. Get professional medical help immediately.

CHEMICAL BURNS

TREATMENT

1. Remove contaminated clothing.
2. Flush burned area with cool water for at least 5 minutes.
3. Treat as you would any major or minor burn.
4. If eye has been burned:
A. Immediately flood face, inside of eyelid and eye with cool running water for at least 15 minutes. Turn head so water does not drain into uninjured eye. Lift eyelid away from eye so the inside of lid can also be washed.
B. If eye has been burned by a dry chemical, lift any loose particles off the eye with the corner of a sterile pad or clean cloth.
C. Cover both eyes with dry sterile pads, clean cloths, or eye pads; bandage in place.
5. Consult professional medical help.

CHOKING, AIRWAY OBSTRUCTION

Partial Obstruction with Good Air Exchange

SYMPTOMS

May include: Forceful cough with wheezing sounds between coughs.

TREATMENT

Encourage victim to cough as long as good air exchange continues. DO NOT interfere with attempts to expel object.

Partial or Complete Airway Obstruction in Conscious Victim with Poor Air Exchange

SYMPTOMS
May include: Weak cough; high-pitched crowing noises during inhalation; inability to breathe, cough or speak; gesture of clutching neck between thumb and index finger; exaggerated breathing efforts; dusky or bluish skin color.

TREATMENT

For Adult Victim If victim is standing or sitting:
1. Stand slightly behind victim.
2. Place your arms around victim's waist; place your fist, thumb side in, against victim's abdomen, slightly above the navel and below the rib margins.
3. Grasp fist with your other hand and exert a quick upward thrust. Repeat (five times in a rapid succession) if necessary (Heimlich Maneuver or manual thrust.)

Complete Airway Obstruction in Unconscious Victim
1. Activate EMS system first. Follow breathing problems section

PENETRATING OBJECTS

Such as Sticks or Pieces of Metal Protruding from Body

SYMPTOMS May include: Profuse bleeding; swelling and redness of injured tissue.

CAUTION DO NOT remove penetrating object.

TREATMENT

1. Get professional medical help immediately.

2A. If victim is fixed to object (impaled), cut it off at a safe distance from skin. Immobilize object with thick dressings made from sterile pads or clean cloths secured in place with first aid tape, a belt or a bandage.

B. If object is protruding from victim, DO NOT move it. Immobilize object with thick dressings made from sterile pads or clean cloths secured in place with first aid tape, a belt or a bandage. Do not apply bandage so tightly that breathing is restricted.

3. If object penetrates chest and victim complains of discomfort or pressure, quickly loosen bandage on one side and reseal. Watch carefully for recurrence. Repeat procedure if necessary.

4. If breathing problems develop, begin rescue breathing techniques immediately.

5. Treat for shock.

POISONING

CALL 911, YOUR LOCAL FIRST AID SQUAD, OR POISON CONTROL CENTER IMMEDIATELY, BEFORE ADMINISTERING FIRST AID.

TREATMENT

1. DO NOT give any other first aid if victim is unconscious or is having convulsions. Begin rescue breathing techniques or CPR if necessary. If victim is convulsing, protect from further injury; loosen tight clothing if possible.

2. If professional medical help cannot be reached immediately:

A. DO NOT induce vomiting if poison is unknown, a corrosive substance (i.e., acid, cleaning fluid, lye, drain cleaner), or a petroleum product (i.e., gasoline, turpentine, paint thinner, lighter fluid). DO NOT use activated charcoal.

B. Induce vomiting if poison is known and is not a corrosive substance or petroleum product. To induce vomiting: Give adult one ounce of syrup of ipecac (1/2 ounce for child) followed by four or five glasses of water. If victim has vomited, follow with one ounce of powdered, activated charcoal in water, if available.

3. Take poison container (or vomitus if poison is unknown) with victim to the hospital.

SEVERED BODY PARTS (AVULSION)

Tissue is Partially or Completely Cut or Torn from Body

CAUTION
Wrap the detached part of the body in something clean, and send it to the hospital with the victim so that it may be reattached if possible. Ice may be used to keep the detached part cool; however, prevent it from direct contact with ice and/or from freezing.

TREATMENT

1. Stop the bleeding immediately.
2. Treat for shock if necessary. If breathing problems are present, begin rescue breathing techniques.
3. If wound is not deep or is not bleeding severely, gently cleanse with mild soap and warm water. Cover with a sterile dressing or clean cloth and bandage.
4. Get professional medical help immediately.

SHOCK

Disturbance in the Circulation of the Blood That Can Upset All Body Functions

CAUTION
Shock is a dangerous condition and can be fatal. Expect some degree of shock in any emergency. DO NOT give anything by mouth.

SYMPTOMS
May include: Unusual weakness or faintness; cold, pale, clammy skin; rapid, weak pulse; shallow, irregular breathing; chills; nausea; unconsciousness.

TREATMENT
1. Treat known cause of shock as quickly as possible (i.e., breathing difficulties, bleeding, severe pain).
2. Maintain an open airway. If victim vomits, gently turn head to side.
3. Keep victim warm and lying flat. (In cases of head or chest injuries, with no chance of broken neck or back, elevate head and shoulders 10 inches higher than feet if possible.)
4. Get professional medical help immediately.
5. DO NOT give anything by mouth.

SPRAINS

Injury to Soft Tissue Surrounding Joint Due to Wrenching or Laceration of Ligaments, Muscles, Tendons or Blood Vessels

SYMPTOMS May include: Painful movement, swelling, discoloration and tenderness around injured joint.

CAUTION
Victim may have a broken bone (fracture) and should be examined by a medical professional.

TREATMENT
1. If ankle or knee is affected, do not allow victim to walk. Loosen or remove shoe; elevate leg.
2. Protect skin with thin towel or cloth. Then apply cold, wet compresses or cold packs to affected area. Never pack joint in ice or immerse in icy water.
3. Consult professional medical assistance for further treatment if necessary.

TRANSPORTING AN INJURED PERSON

If injury involves neck or back, DO NOT move victim unless absolutely necessary. Call for professional medical help.

If victim must be pulled to safety, move body lengthwise, not sideways. If possible, slide a coat or blanket under the victim:

A. Carefully turn victim toward you and slip a half-rolled blanket under back.

B. Turn victim on side over blanket, unroll, and return victim onto back.

C. Drag victim head first, keeping back as straight as possible.

If victim must be lifted:

A. Support each part of the body. Position a person at victim's head to provide additional stability. Use a board, shutter, table top or other firm surface to keep body as level as possible.

UNCONSCIOUSNESS

Victim Is Not Mentally Aware; Does Not Respond to Sensory Stimuli, Such as Sound or Light

TREATMENT
1. Call for professional medical help.
2. DO NOT move victim or give anything by mouth.
3. Keep victim warm; loosen any tight clothing.
4. Maintain an open airway. If breathing difficulties develop, begin rescue breathing techniques immediately.
5. Check for emergency medical identification tag to help determine cause of unconsciousness.

WOUNDS (SEVERE)

Breaks in Skin or Mucus Membrane (Open) or Injuries to Underlying Tissue Breaks in Skin (Closed)

CAUTION

Some wounds, such as small cuts or minor scrapes, require only simple first aid measures; others, however, require immediate first aid followed by professional medical treatment. Before treating any serious incision, abrasion or laceration with extensive bleeding, act quickly to control bleeding. Get professional medical help immediately. Any wound can become contaminated and infected.

COLD EXPOSURE

TREATMENT

1. Move victim into warm room as soon as possible.
2. Be alert for breathing difficulties; start rescue breathing techniques if necessary.
3. Remove wet or frozen clothing. Immediately rewarm victim by wrapping in hlankets or placing in tub
of warm, not hot, water. Dry victim thoroughly after bath.
4. Give victim hot liquids to drink, only if conscious (not alcohol).
5. Follow treatment for frostbite.
6. Consult professional medical help if indicated.

FROSTBITE

CAUTION

DO NOT break blisters, rub affected area, or apply heat lamps or hot water bottles. DO NOT attempt rapid thawing if refreezing is a possibility.

TREATMENT

1. Warm affected areas as quickly as possible by covering with clothing and blankets or immersing frozen part in warm, not hot, water. If frostbitten area has been thawed and refrozen, then warm at room temperature.
2. Discontinue warming techniques as soon as affected area becomes flushed. Expect swelling and pain after thawing. Victim may require an analgesic.
3. Gently exercise affected area after it has been rewarmed.
4. DO NOT apply dressings or clothing unless transportation is required for medical help. If fingers or toes are affected, separate with sterile pads or clean cloths.
5. Elevate frostbitten areas, but not higher than heart.
6. Get professional medical help.

HEAT EXHAUSTION

(Heat Prostration)

SYMPTOMS

May include: Fatigue; irritability; headache; faintness; weak, rapid pulse; shallow breathing; cold, clammy skin; profuse perspiration.

TREATMENT

1. Instruct victim to lie down in a cool, shaded area or an air-conditioned room. Elevate feet.
2. Massage legs toward heart.
3. Only if victim is conscious, give cool water or electrolyte solution every 15 minutes until victim recovers.
4. Use caution when letting victim first sit up, even after feeling recovered.

SUNBURN

TREATMENT

1. Treat for first or second degree burns.
2. Treat for shock if necessary.
3. Cool victim as rapidly as possible by applying cool, damp cloths or immersing in cool, not cold, water.
4. Give victim fluids to drink.
5. Get professional medical help immediately for severe cases.

SUNSTROKE

(Heat Stroke)

SYMPTOMS

May include: Extremely high body temperature (106°F or higher); hot, red, dry skin; absence of sweating; rapid pulse; convulsions; unconsciousness.

CAUTION

Sunstroke is a life-threatening emergency.

TREATMENT

1. Get professional medical help immediately.
2. Lower body temperature quickly by placing victim in partially filled tub of cool, not cold, water (avoid over-cooling). Briskly sponge victim's body until temperature is reduced; then towel dry. If tub is not available, wrap victim in cold, wet sheets in well-ventilated room or use fans and air conditioners until body temperature is reduced.
3. DO NOT give stimulating beverages, such as coffee, tea, or soda.